AUTO-IMMUNE IMMUNE PLANT-BASED COOKBOOK

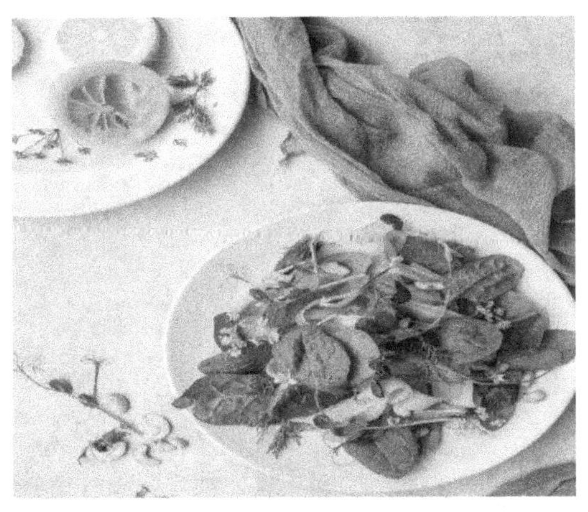

DR. JESSICA SMITH

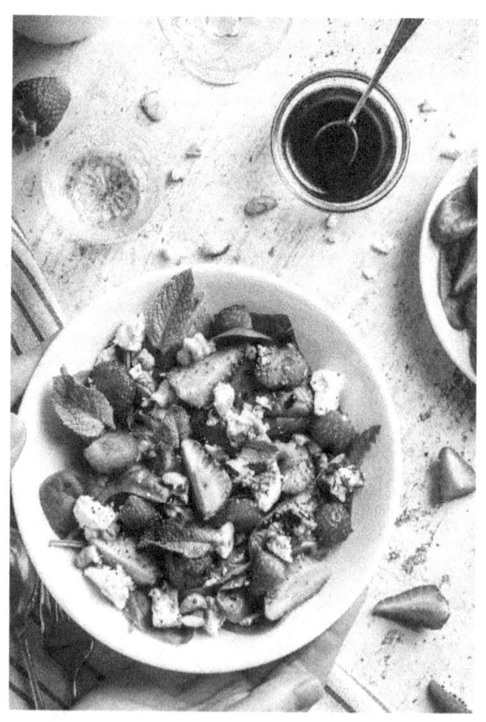

TABLE OF CONTENTS

CHAPTER ONE

How to Use this Cookbook

Identify Your Target Audience: Determine who your cookbook is for. Are you targeting individuals with specific autoimmune conditions like rheumatoid arthritis or lupus? Understanding your audience will help tailor your recipes and content to their needs.

Research Autoimmune-Friendly Foods: Investigate which plant-based foods are beneficial for managing autoimmune conditions. Focus on ingredients that are anti-inflammatory, nutrient-dense, and support gut health, such as leafy greens, berries, turmeric, ginger, and healthy fats like avocado and nuts.

Develop Recipe Categories: Organize your cookbook into categories that cater to different meal times and preferences, such as breakfast, lunch, dinner, snacks, and desserts. Consider including sections for smoothies, salads, soups, main dishes, and healthy treats.

Create Flavorful Recipes: Experiment with flavorful herbs, spices, and seasoning blends to enhance the taste of your dishes. Use ingredients like garlic, basil, cilantro, cumin, and smoked paprika to add depth and complexity to your plant based creations.

Focus on Nutrient Density: Emphasize recipes that are rich in vitamins, minerals, antioxidants, and phytonutrients to support overall health and immune function. Incorporate a variety of colorful fruits and vegetables to ensure a broad spectrum of nutrients.

Include Balanced Meals: Ensure that each recipe provides a balance of macronutrients (carbohydrates, protein, and fats) to support sustained energy levels and satiety. Aim for a combination of whole grains, legumes, vegetables, and plant-based protein sources like tofu, tempeh, or beans in your recipes.

Provide Allergy-Friendly Options: Consider dietary restrictions and allergies commonly associated with autoimmune conditions, such as gluten, dairy, and soy intolerances. Offer alternative ingredients and substitutions to accommodate various dietary needs.

Offer Meal Prep Tips: Include practical meal prep tips and batch cooking suggestions to help readers streamline their cooking process and make healthy eating more convenient. Provide guidance on storing, reheating, and freezing meals for later use.

Incorporate Educational Content: Supplement your recipes with educational content on autoimmune conditions, the role of nutrition in managing symptoms, and lifestyle factors that can support immune health. Include tips on stress management, sleep hygiene, and physical activity.

Provide Testimonials and Success Stories: Share testimonials and success stories from individuals who have benefited from following a plant-based diet to manage their autoimmune condition. Personal anecdotes can inspire and motivate readers to adopt healthier dietary habits.

By following these 10 easy steps, you can create a comprehensive Auto-Immune Plant-Based Cookbook that empowers individuals with autoimmune conditions to nourish their bodies with delicious and nutritious plant-based meals.

Understanding Auto-Immune Plant Based

Understanding Auto-Immune Plant-Based eating involves recognizing the intricate relationship between diet and autoimmune conditions, where the immune system mistakenly attacks healthy cells.

A plant-based approach to eating emphasizes whole, minimally processed foods derived from plants, such as fruits, vegetables, grains, legumes, nuts, and seeds.

This dietary approach aims to reduce inflammation, support gut health, and provide essential nutrients that may help manage autoimmune symptoms.

Plant-based diets are rich in antioxidants, phytonutrients, vitamins, and minerals, which can help modulate the immune response and promote overall well-being.

By avoiding animal products and highly processed foods, individuals following an autoimmune plant-based diet may reduce exposure to potential triggers and allergens commonly associated with autoimmune conditions.

Moreover, plant-based eating emphasizes foods that are naturally anti-inflammatory, such as leafy greens, berries, turmeric, ginger, and omega-3 fatty acids found in walnuts, flaxseeds, and chia seeds.

These foods may help alleviate symptoms like joint pain, fatigue, and inflammation commonly experienced by individuals with autoimmune disorders.

Understanding the principles of Auto-Immune Plant-Based eating involves not only choosing the right foods but also adopting a holistic approach to health that encompasses stress management, adequate sleep, regular physical activity, and mindful eating practices.

By embracing a plant-based lifestyle, individuals with autoimmune conditions can nourish their bodies with nutrient-dense foods that support immune function and promote long-term wellness.

Principles of Auto-Immune Plant Based

The principles of Auto-Immune Plant-Based eating revolve around nourishing the body with nutrient-dense plant foods while minimizing potential triggers and inflammatory agents that may exacerbate autoimmune symptoms.

These principles are rooted in the understanding that certain plant-based foods possess anti-inflammatory, antioxidant, and immune-modulating properties that can support overall health and potentially alleviate autoimmune-related symptoms.

One principle of Auto-Immune Plant-Based eating is to prioritize whole, unprocessed plant foods.

This includes fruits, vegetables, whole grains, legumes, nuts, and seeds, which are abundant in vitamins, minerals, fiber, and phytonutrients.

These nutrient-rich foods help to reduce inflammation and provide essential nutrients necessary for immune function and overall well-being.

Another principle is to focus on diversity and variety in food choices.

Consuming a wide range of plant-based foods ensures that individuals receive a spectrum of nutrients and antioxidants that can help support immune health and reduce the risk of nutrient deficiencies commonly associated with autoimmune conditions.

Additionally, Auto-Immune Plant-Based eating emphasizes the importance of avoiding or minimizing inflammatory foods, such as processed foods, refined sugars, artificial additives, and certain oils.

These substances have been linked to increased inflammation and may exacerbate autoimmune symptoms in some individuals.

Furthermore, incorporating plant-based sources of omega-3 fatty acids, such as flaxseeds, chia seeds, walnuts, and hemp seeds, is encouraged.

Omega-3 fatty acids have anti-inflammatory properties and may help reduce inflammation associated with autoimmune conditions.

Benefits of Auto-Immune Plant Based

The benefits of Auto-Immune Plant-Based eating extend beyond mere nutrition, offering a holistic approach to managing autoimmune conditions and promoting overall health and well-being.

One significant advantage is the potential reduction of inflammation throughout the body.

Plant-based diets are naturally rich in anti-inflammatory compounds such as antioxidants, phytonutrients, and fiber, which can help mitigate chronic inflammation associated with autoimmune disorders. By reducing inflammation, individuals may experience relief from symptoms such as joint pain, fatigue, and gastrointestinal discomfort.

Moreover, Auto-Immune Plant-Based eating emphasizes foods that support gut health, which is closely linked to immune function.

Plant-based diets are high in fiber, prebiotics, and beneficial plant compounds that nourish gut bacteria and promote a healthy microbiome.

A balanced gut microbiome is essential for regulating immune responses and reducing autoimmune flare-ups.

Another benefit is the potential improvement in overall nutrient intake. Plant-based diets are abundant in vitamins, minerals, and phytonutrients, which are essential for immune function and overall health.

By consuming a variety of plant foods, individuals can ensure they receive adequate nutrients to support their bodies' needs and potentially reduce the risk of nutrient deficiencies common in autoimmune conditions.

Additionally, adopting a plant-based lifestyle may lead to better weight management and cardiovascular health.

Plant-based diets are generally lower in saturated fats and cholesterol and higher in fiber and healthy fats, which can help lower cholesterol levels, improve blood sugar control, and support heart health.

Tips for Auto-Immune Plant Based

Transitioning to an Auto-Immune Plant-Based diet can be a transformative journey towards managing autoimmune conditions effectively while embracing a healthier lifestyle. Here are some helpful tips to navigate this dietary shift:

Educate Yourself: Take the time to learn about Auto-Immune Plant-Based eating, including which foods are beneficial and which to avoid. Understand the principles behind this dietary approach to make informed choices.

Start Slowly: Gradually incorporate more plant-based foods into your diet and experiment with new recipes. This gradual approach can help your taste buds adapt and make the transition smoother.

Focus on Whole Foods: Emphasize whole, minimally processed plant foods such as fruits, vegetables, whole grains, legumes, nuts, and seeds. These nutrient-dense foods provide essential vitamins, minerals, and antioxidants to support immune health.

Experiment with Recipes: Get creative in the kitchen and explore different ways to prepare plant-based meals. Try new cooking techniques, spices, and flavor combinations to keep your meals interesting and enjoyable.

Plan Ahead: Plan your meals and snacks in advance to ensure you have nutritious options readily available. Batch cooking and meal prepping can save time and make it easier to stick to your dietary goals.

Listen to Your Body: Pay attention to how different foods make you feel and adjust your diet accordingly. Keep a food journal to track your symptoms and identify any potential triggers.

Stay Hydrated: Drink plenty of water throughout the day to support digestion, detoxification, and overall health.

Seek Support: Connect with others following a similar dietary approach for support, advice, and recipe ideas.

Online forums, social media groups, and local meetups can be valuable resources.

Be Patient and Persistent: Remember that transitioning to a new way of eating takes time and effort. Be patient with yourself and stay committed to your health goals.

Consult a Healthcare Professional: If you have specific dietary concerns or medical conditions, consult with a registered dietitian or healthcare provider before making significant changes to your diet.

By incorporating these tips into your journey, you can successfully adopt an Auto-Immune Plant-Based diet and reap the many health benefits it has to offer.

Guidelines for Auto-Immune Plant Based

Following guidelines for an Auto-Immune Plant-Based diet can help individuals effectively manage autoimmune conditions while promoting overall health and well-being. Here are some key guidelines to consider:

Emphasize Whole Foods: Focus on consuming a variety of whole, minimally processed plant foods such as fruits, vegetables, whole grains, legumes, nuts, and seeds.

These foods are rich in nutrients, fiber, and antioxidants that support immune health and reduce inflammation.

Prioritize Anti-Inflammatory Foods: Include foods that are known for their anti-inflammatory properties, such as berries, leafy greens, turmeric, ginger, and omega-3 fatty acids found in flaxseeds, chia seeds, and walnuts. These foods can help alleviate autoimmune symptoms and promote overall well-being.

Avoid Trigger Foods: Identify and eliminate potential trigger foods that may exacerbate autoimmune symptoms. Common trigger foods include gluten, dairy, soy, processed sugars, and artificial additives. Pay attention to how your body reacts to certain foods and adjust your diet accordingly.

Optimize Gut Health: Support gut health by consuming foods rich in fiber, prebiotics, and probiotics. These include fruits, vegetables, whole grains, fermented foods like sauerkraut and kimchi, and probiotic-rich foods like yogurt and kefir. A healthy gut microbiome is essential for regulating immune function and reducing inflammation.

Stay Hydrated: Drink plenty of water throughout the day to stay hydrated and support overall health.

Hydration is important for digestion, detoxification, and maintaining optimal bodily functions.

Practice Mindful Eating: Eat mindfully, paying attention to hunger and fullness cues, and savoring each bite. Avoid distractions while eating and take the time to enjoy your meals.

Include Healthy Fats: Incorporate sources of healthy fats into your diet, such as avocados, nuts, seeds, and olive oil. These fats provide essential fatty acids and support brain health, hormone balance, and inflammation reduction.

Supplement Wisely: Consider supplementing your diet with nutrients that may be lacking, such as vitamin D, vitamin B12, omega-3 fatty acids, and probiotics. Consult with a healthcare professional to determine which supplements are appropriate for you.

Monitor Symptom Response: Pay attention to how your body responds to different foods and adjust your diet accordingly. Keep a food journal to track your symptoms and identify potential triggers.

Seek Professional Guidance: Consult with a registered dietitian or healthcare provider who specializes in autoimmune conditions and plant-based nutrition. They can provide personalized guidance and support to help you optimize your diet for managing autoimmune symptoms effectively.

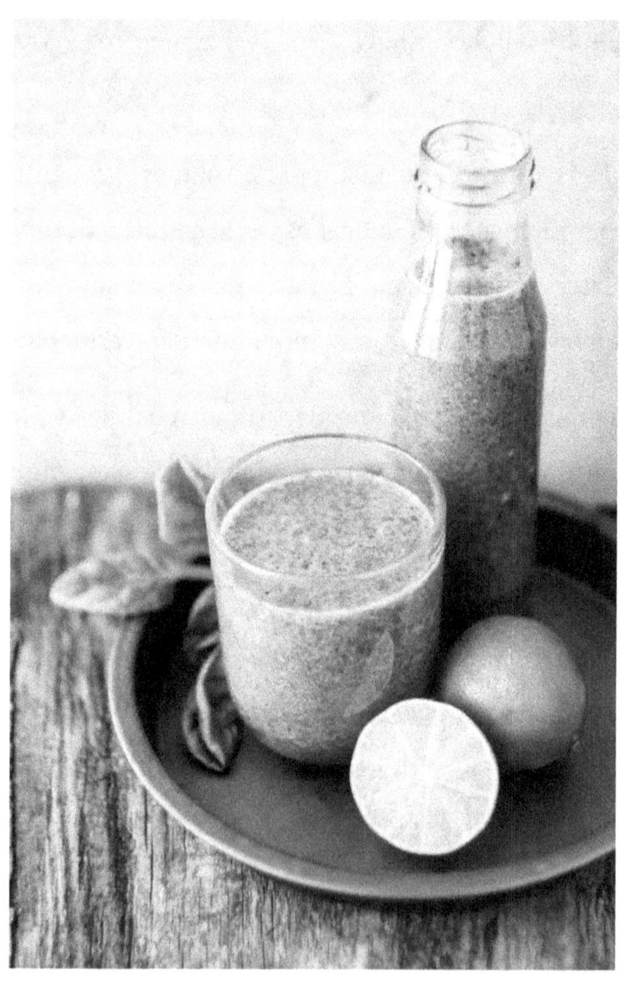

CHAPTER TWO

Auto-Immune Plant Based Recipes

1. Turmeric Lentil Soup

Ingredients:

- ➢ 1 cup red lentils, rinsed
- ➢ 4 cups vegetable broth
- ➢ 1 onion, diced
- ➢ 2 carrots, diced
- ➢ 2 celery stalks, diced
- ➢ 2 cloves garlic, minced
- ➢ 1 tablespoon turmeric powder
- ➢ 1 teaspoon ground cumin
- ➢ 1 teaspoon ground coriander
- ➢ Salt and pepper to taste
- ➢ Fresh cilantro for garnish (optional)

Instructions:

- ➢ In a large pot, sauté onions, carrots, and celery until softened.
- ➢ Add minced garlic, turmeric, cumin, and coriander. Cook for 1-2 minutes until fragrant.

- ➢ Add rinsed lentils and vegetable broth. Bring to a boil, then reduce heat and simmer for 20-25 minutes, or until lentils are tender.
- ➢ Season with salt and pepper to taste. Serve hot, garnished with fresh cilantro if desired.

Health Benefits:

- ➢ Turmeric is anti-inflammatory and may help alleviate autoimmune symptoms.
- ➢ Lentils are rich in protein, fiber, and iron.
- ➢ Vegetables provide essential vitamins and minerals for immune support.

Preparation Time: 30 minutes

2. Quinoa Stuffed Bell Peppers

Ingredients:

- ➢ 4 large bell peppers, halved and seeds removed
- ➢ 1 cup quinoa, rinsed
- ➢ 2 cups vegetable broth
- ➢ 1 onion, diced
- ➢ 2 cloves garlic, minced
- ➢ 1 cup diced tomatoes

- ➢ 1 cup black beans, drained and rinsed
- ➢ 1 teaspoon cumin
- ➢ 1 teaspoon paprika
- ➢ Salt and pepper to taste
- ➢ Fresh parsley for garnish (optional)

Instructions:

- ➢ Preheat oven to 375°F (190°C).
- ➢ In a saucepan, combine quinoa and vegetable broth. Bring to a boil, then reduce heat and simmer for 15-20 minutes, or until quinoa is cooked.
- ➢ In a skillet, sauté onions and garlic until softened. Add diced tomatoes, black beans, cumin, paprika, salt, and pepper. Cook for another 5 minutes.
- ➢ Stir cooked quinoa into the skillet mixture.
- ➢ Stuff bell pepper halves with quinoa mixture and place them in a baking dish.
- ➢ Cover with foil and bake for 25-30 minutes, or until peppers are tender.
- ➢ Garnish with fresh parsley before serving.

Health Benefits: Quinoa is a complete protein source and gluten-free grain.

> Bell peppers are rich in vitamin C and antioxidants.

> Black beans provide fiber and plant-based protein.

Preparation Time: 50 minutes

3. Roasted Vegetable Buddha Bowl

Ingredients:

> 1 cup cooked quinoa or brown rice

> 1 sweet potato, diced

> 1 cup broccoli florets

> 1 cup cauliflower florets

> 1 tablespoon olive oil

> 1 teaspoon garlic powder

> 1 teaspoon paprika

> Salt and pepper to taste

> Tahini dressing (optional)

Instructions:

> Preheat oven to 400°F (200°C).

> Toss diced sweet potato, broccoli, and cauliflower with olive oil, garlic powder, paprika, salt, and pepper on a baking sheet.

- Roast vegetables for 20-25 minutes, or until tender and lightly browned.
- Divide cooked quinoa or brown rice among serving bowls.
- Top with roasted vegetables.
- Drizzle with tahini dressing if desired.

Health Benefits:

- Sweet potatoes are rich in beta-carotene and vitamin A.
- Broccoli and cauliflower are cruciferous vegetables that support detoxification.
- Quinoa and brown rice provide complex carbohydrates for sustained energy.

Preparation Time: 30 minutes

4. Chickpea Spinach Curry

Ingredients:

- 1 tablespoon coconut oil
- 1 onion, diced
- 2 cloves garlic, minced
- 1 tablespoon ginger, grated

- 1 tablespoon curry powder
- 1 teaspoon ground turmeric
- 1 can (15 oz) chickpeas, drained and rinsed
- 1 can (14 oz) diced tomatoes
- 1 cup coconut milk
- 2 cups baby spinach
- Salt and pepper to taste
- Fresh cilantro for garnish (optional)

Instructions:

- In a large skillet, heat coconut oil over medium heat. Add diced onion and cook until translucent.
- Add minced garlic and grated ginger. Cook for another minute until fragrant.
- Stir in curry powder and turmeric.
- Add chickpeas, diced tomatoes, and coconut milk. Simmer for 10-15 minutes.
- Stir in baby spinach and cook until wilted.
- Season with salt and pepper to taste.
- Garnish with fresh cilantro before serving.

Health Benefits: Chickpeas are a good source of plant-based protein and fiber.

➤ Spinach is rich in iron and vitamin C.

➤ Turmeric and ginger have anti-inflammatory properties.

Preparation Time: 25 minutes

5. Butternut Squash Soup

Ingredients:

➤ 1 butternut squash, peeled, seeded, and cubed

➤ 1 onion, diced

➤ 2 carrots, diced

➤ 2 cloves garlic, minced

➤ 4 cups vegetable broth

➤ 1 teaspoon ground cinnamon

➤ 1/2 teaspoon ground nutmeg

➤ Salt and pepper to taste

➤ Coconut cream for garnish (optional)

Instructions:

➤ In a large pot, sauté diced onion and carrots until softened.

➤ Add minced garlic and cook for another minute.

- Add cubed butternut squash and vegetable broth. Bring to a boil, then reduce heat and simmer for 20-25 minutes, or until squash is tender.
- Use an immersion blender to puree the soup until smooth. Alternatively, transfer the soup to a blender and blend until smooth.
- Stir in ground cinnamon and nutmeg. Season with salt and pepper to taste.
- Serve hot, garnished with a drizzle of coconut cream if desired.

Health Benefits:

- Butternut squash is rich in vitamins A and C.
- Carrots provide beta-carotene, which supports immune health.
- Cinnamon and nutmeg add warmth and flavor.

Preparation Time: 40 minutes

6. Rainbow Veggie Stir-Fry

Ingredients:

- 1 cup cooked quinoa or brown rice
- 1 tablespoon sesame oil

- ➢ 1 onion, sliced
- ➢ 2 cloves garlic, minced
- ➢ 1 bell pepper, sliced
- ➢ 1 cup broccoli florets
- ➢ 1 cup shredded cabbage
- ➢ 1 carrot, julienned
- ➢ 1 cup mushrooms, sliced
- ➢ 2 tablespoons tamari or soy sauce
- ➢ 1 tablespoon rice vinegar
- ➢ 1 teaspoon grated ginger
- ➢ Sesame seeds for garnish (optional)

Instructions:

- ➢ Heat sesame oil in a large skillet or wok over medium-high heat.
- ➢ Add sliced onion and minced garlic. Stir-fry for 2-3 minutes until fragrant.
- ➢ Add bell pepper, broccoli, cabbage, carrot, and mushrooms to the skillet. Stir-fry for another 5-7 minutes until vegetables are tender-crisp.
- ➢ In a small bowl, whisk together tamari or soy sauce, rice vinegar, and grated ginger.

- Pour the sauce over the vegetables and stir to coat evenly.
- Serve stir-fried vegetables over cooked quinoa or brown rice.
- Garnish with sesame seeds before serving.

Health Benefits:

- Colorful vegetables provide a variety of vitamins, minerals, and antioxidants.
- Quinoa and brown rice offer complex carbohydrates and protein for sustained energy.
- Ginger may help reduce inflammation and aid digestion.

Preparation Time: 25 minutes

7. Beet and Lentil Salad

Ingredients:

- 1 cup cooked green lentils
- 2 medium beets, roasted, peeled, and diced
- 1/4 cup chopped fresh parsley
- 2 tablespoons olive oil
- 1 tablespoon balsamic vinegar

- ➤ 1 tablespoon maple syrup

- ➤ Salt and pepper to taste

- ➤ 1/4 cup chopped walnuts for garnish (optional)

Instructions:

- ➤ In a large bowl, combine cooked green lentils, diced roasted beets, and chopped fresh parsley.

- ➤ In a small bowl, whisk together olive oil, balsamic vinegar, maple syrup, salt, and pepper to make the dressing.

- ➤ Pour the dressing over the lentil and beet mixture. Toss to coat evenly.

- ➤ Garnish with chopped walnuts before serving.

Health Benefits:

- ➤ Lentils are a good source of plant-based protein and fiber.

- ➤ Beets are rich in antioxidants and may help reduce inflammation.

- ➤ Walnuts provide omega-3 fatty acids and add crunch.

Preparation Time: 30 minutes (including roasting time for beets)

8. Spinach and Mushroom Quinoa Bowl

Ingredients:

- 1 cup cooked quinoa
- 2 cups baby spinach
- 1 cup sliced mushrooms
- 1 clove garlic, minced
- 1 tablespoon olive oil
- 1 tablespoon lemon juice
- Salt and pepper to taste
- Hemp seeds for garnish (optional)

Instructions:

- Heat olive oil in a skillet over medium heat. Add minced garlic and sliced mushrooms. Cook for 5-7 minutes until mushrooms are golden brown.
- Add baby spinach to the skillet and cook until wilted.
- Stir in cooked quinoa and lemon juice. Season with salt and pepper to taste.
- Serve quinoa mixture in bowls, garnished with hemp seeds if desired.

Health Benefits: Quinoa provides protein, fiber, and essential amino acids.

- ➤ Spinach is rich in iron and vitamins A and C.
- ➤ Mushrooms contain immune-boosting compounds like beta-glucans.

Preparation Time: 20 minutes

9. Cauliflower Rice Sushi Rolls

Ingredients:

- ➤ 1 head cauliflower, riced
- ➤ 2 tablespoons rice vinegar
- ➤ 1 tablespoon maple syrup
- ➤ Salt to taste
- ➤ Nori sheets
- ➤ Assorted thinly sliced vegetables (cucumber, avocado, bell pepper, carrot)
- ➤ Pickled ginger, wasabi, and soy sauce for serving

Instructions:

- ➤ In a large bowl, combine riced cauliflower, rice vinegar, maple syrup, and salt. Mix well to combine.
- ➤ Place a nori sheet on a bamboo sushi mat. Spread a thin layer of cauliflower rice evenly over the nori sheet, leaving a small border around the edges.

- ➢ Arrange thinly sliced vegetables in the center of the cauliflower rice.
- ➢ Using the bamboo sushi mat, tightly roll the nori sheet into a sushi roll.
- ➢ Slice the sushi roll into bite-sized pieces using a sharp knife.
- ➢ Serve sushi rolls with pickled ginger, wasabi, and soy sauce for dipping.

Health Benefits:

- ➢ Cauliflower rice is low in carbohydrates and rich in vitamins C and K.
- ➢ Nori sheets provide iodine, essential for thyroid health.
- ➢ Assorted vegetables add fiber, vitamins, and minerals.

Preparation Time: 30 minutes

10. Berry Chia Seed Pudding

Ingredients:

- ➢ 1/4 cup chia seeds
- ➢ 1 cup unsweetened almond milk

- ➢ 1 tablespoon maple syrup
- ➢ 1/2 teaspoon vanilla extract
- ➢ Assorted berries for topping (strawberries, blueberries, raspberries)

Instructions:

- ➢ In a bowl, whisk together chia seeds, almond milk, maple syrup, and vanilla extract.
- ➢ Cover and refrigerate for at least 2 hours or overnight, until the mixture thickens into a pudding-like consistency.
- ➢ Stir the chia seed pudding to redistribute the seeds evenly.
- ➢ Serve chilled, topped with assorted berries.

Health Benefits:

- ➢ Chia seeds are rich in omega-3 fatty acids, fiber, and antioxidants.
- ➢ Berries provide vitamins, minerals, and antioxidants.
- ➢ Maple syrup adds natural sweetness without refined sugars.

Preparation Time: 5 minutes (plus chilling time)

11. Sweet Potato and Kale Hash

Ingredients:

- ➢ 2 large sweet potatoes, peeled and diced
- ➢ 1 bunch kale, stems removed and leaves chopped
- ➢ 1 onion, diced
- ➢ 2 cloves garlic, minced
- ➢ 1 tablespoon olive oil
- ➢ 1 teaspoon smoked paprika
- ➢ Salt and pepper to taste
- ➢ Fresh parsley for garnish (optional)

Instructions:

- ➢ Heat olive oil in a skillet over medium heat. Add diced sweet potatoes and cook until tender, about 10 minutes.
- ➢ Add diced onion and minced garlic to the skillet. Cook for another 5 minutes until onions are translucent.
- ➢ Stir in chopped kale and smoked paprika. Cook until kale is wilted.
- ➢ Season with salt and pepper to taste. Garnish with fresh parsley before serving.

Health Benefits:

- ➢ Sweet potatoes are rich in beta-carotene and vitamin A.
- ➢ Kale is packed with vitamins K, A, and C, as well as antioxidants.
- ➢ Olive oil provides healthy fats and adds flavor.

Preparation Time: 25 minutes

12. Lentil and Vegetable Shepherd's Pie

Ingredients:

- ➢ 2 cups cooked green lentils
- ➢ 1 onion, diced
- ➢ 2 carrots, diced
- ➢ 2 celery stalks, diced
- ➢ 2 cloves garlic, minced
- ➢ 1 cup frozen peas
- ➢ 1 tablespoon tomato paste
- ➢ 1 cup vegetable broth
- ➢ 2 tablespoons olive oil
- ➢ Salt and pepper to taste
- ➢ Mashed sweet potatoes for topping

Instructions:

- ➤ Preheat oven to 375°F (190°C).
- ➤ Heat olive oil in a skillet over medium heat. Add diced onion, carrots, celery, and minced garlic. Cook until vegetables are softened.
- ➤ Stir in cooked green lentils, frozen peas, tomato paste, and vegetable broth. Cook for another 5 minutes.
- ➤ Transfer the lentil and vegetable mixture to a baking dish. Spread mashed sweet potatoes evenly over the top.
- ➤ Bake for 20-25 minutes, or until the sweet potato topping is golden brown.
- ➤ Serve hot.

Health Benefits:

- ➤ Lentils are rich in protein, fiber, and iron.
- ➤ Vegetables provide essential vitamins, minerals, and antioxidants.
- ➤ Sweet potatoes add sweetness and nutrients.

Preparation Time: 45 minutes

13. Almond Butter Banana Smoothie

Ingredients:

> - 1 ripe banana
> - 2 tablespoons almond butter
> - 1 cup unsweetened almond milk
> - 1 tablespoon chia seeds
> - 1 teaspoon cinnamon
> - Ice cubes (optional)

Instructions:

> - Combine all ingredients in a blender.
> - Blend until smooth and creamy.
> - Add ice cubes if desired for a colder smoothie.
> - Pour into glasses and serve immediately.

Health Benefits:

> - Bananas are rich in potassium and provide natural sweetness.
> - Almond butter adds healthy fats and protein.
> - Chia seeds provide omega-3 fatty acids and fiber.

Preparation Time: 5 minutes

14. Mediterranean Quinoa Salad

Ingredients:

- ➢ 1 cup cooked quinoa
- ➢ 1 cup cherry tomatoes, halved
- ➢ 1 cucumber, diced
- ➢ 1/2 red onion, thinly sliced
- ➢ 1/4 cup Kalamata olives, sliced
- ➢ 1/4 cup chopped fresh parsley
- ➢ 2 tablespoons extra virgin olive oil
- ➢ 1 tablespoon lemon juice
- ➢ 1 teaspoon dried oregano
- ➢ Salt and pepper to taste

Instructions:

- ➢ In a large bowl, combine cooked quinoa, cherry tomatoes, cucumber, red onion, Kalamata olives, and chopped fresh parsley.
- ➢ In a small bowl, whisk together extra virgin olive oil, lemon juice, dried oregano, salt, and pepper to make the dressing.
- ➢ Pour the dressing over the quinoa salad and toss to combine.

➢ Serve chilled or at room temperature.

Health Benefits:

➢ Quinoa provides protein, fiber, and essential amino acids.

➢ Cherry tomatoes and cucumber add hydration and vitamins.

➢ Olives and olive oil offer healthy fats and antioxidants.

Preparation Time: 20 minutes

15. Cauliflower and Broccoli Soup

Ingredients:

➢ 1 head cauliflower, chopped

➢ 2 cups broccoli florets

➢ 1 onion, diced

➢ 2 cloves garlic, minced

➢ 4 cups vegetable broth

➢ 1/2 cup coconut milk

➢ 1 tablespoon nutritional yeast (optional)

➢ Salt and pepper to taste

➢ Fresh chives for garnish (optional)

Instructions:

> - In a large pot, sauté diced onion and minced garlic until softened.
> - Add chopped cauliflower, broccoli florets, and vegetable broth to the pot. Bring to a boil, then reduce heat and simmer for 15-20 minutes, or until vegetables are tender.
> - Use an immersion blender to puree the soup until smooth. Alternatively, transfer the soup to a blender and blend until smooth.
> - Stir in coconut milk and nutritional yeast, if using. Season with salt and pepper to taste.
> - Serve hot, garnished with fresh chives if desired.

Health Benefits:

> - Cauliflower and broccoli are cruciferous vegetables that support detoxification.
> - Coconut milk adds creaminess and healthy fats.
> - Nutritional yeast provides a cheesy flavor and is rich in B vitamins.

Preparation Time: 30 minutes

16. Avocado and White Bean Salad

Ingredients:

- ➢ 1 can (15 oz) white beans, drained and rinsed
- ➢ 1 avocado, diced
- ➢ 1 cup cherry tomatoes, halved
- ➢ 1/4 cup red onion, diced
- ➢ 2 tablespoons chopped fresh cilantro
- ➢ 1 tablespoon extra virgin olive oil
- ➢ 1 tablespoon lime juice
- ➢ Salt and pepper to taste

Instructions:

- ➢ In a large bowl, combine white beans, diced avocado, cherry tomatoes, diced red onion, and chopped fresh cilantro.
- ➢ In a small bowl, whisk together extra virgin olive oil, lime juice, salt, and pepper to make the dressing.
- ➢ Pour the dressing over the bean salad and toss to coat evenly.
- ➢ Serve chilled or at room temperature.

Health Benefits: White beans provide plant-based protein and fiber.

- ➢ Avocado adds healthy fats and creaminess.
- ➢ Cherry tomatoes and red onion add color, flavor, and nutrients.

Preparation Time: 15 minutes

17. Spaghetti Squash Primavera

Ingredients:

- ➢ 1 large spaghetti squash
- ➢ 2 tablespoons olive oil
- ➢ 2 cloves garlic, minced
- ➢ 1 cup cherry tomatoes, halved
- ➢ 1 cup broccoli florets
- ➢ 1/2 cup diced bell pepper
- ➢ 1/4 cup chopped fresh basil
- ➢ Salt and pepper to taste
- ➢ Vegan Parmesan cheese for garnish (optional)

Instructions:

- ➢ Preheat oven to 400°F (200°C).
- ➢ Cut spaghetti squash in half lengthwise and scoop out the seeds.

- Place spaghetti squash halves, cut side down, on a baking sheet. Bake for 40-45 minutes, or until squash is tender.
- While the squash is baking, heat olive oil in a skillet over medium heat. Add minced garlic and cook for 1-2 minutes until fragrant.
- Add cherry tomatoes, broccoli florets, and diced bell pepper to the skillet. Cook for 5-7 minutes until vegetables are tender-crisp.
- Use a fork to scrape the spaghetti squash strands into the skillet with the cooked vegetables.
- Stir in chopped fresh basil. Season with salt and pepper to taste.
- Serve hot, garnished with vegan Parmesan cheese if desired.

Health Benefits:

- Spaghetti squash is low in calories and carbohydrates.
- Cherry tomatoes, broccoli, and bell pepper provide vitamins, minerals, and antioxidants.
- Basil adds flavor and is rich in vitamin K.

Preparation Time: 60 minutes

18. Apple Cinnamon Oatmeal

Ingredients:

- 1 cup rolled oats
- 2 cups unsweetened almond milk
- 1 apple, diced
- 1 tablespoon maple syrup
- 1 teaspoon ground cinnamon
- 1/4 teaspoon ground nutmeg
- 1/4 cup chopped walnuts
- Fresh apple slices for garnish (optional)

Instructions:

- In a saucepan, combine rolled oats, almond milk, diced apple, maple syrup, ground cinnamon, and ground nutmeg.
- Bring the mixture to a boil, then reduce heat and simmer for 5-7 minutes, stirring occasionally, until oats are cooked and the mixture thickens.
- Remove from heat and stir in chopped walnuts.
- Serve hot, garnished with fresh apple slices if desired.

Health Benefits:

- Oats are a good source of soluble fiber and may help lower cholesterol levels.
- Apples provide fiber, vitamin C, and antioxidants.
- Cinnamon adds warmth and may help regulate blood sugar levels.

Preparation Time: 10 minutes

19. Mediterranean Chickpea Salad

Ingredients:

- 1 can (15 oz) chickpeas, drained and rinsed
- 1 cucumber, diced
- 1 bell pepper, diced
- 1/4 cup red onion, diced
- 1/4 cup Kalamata olives, sliced
- 2 tablespoons chopped fresh parsley
- 2 tablespoons extra virgin olive oil
- 1 tablespoon lemon juice
- 1 teaspoon dried oregano
- Salt and pepper to taste

Instructions:

> ➤ In a large bowl, combine chickpeas, diced cucumber, diced bell pepper, diced red onion, sliced Kalamata olives, and chopped fresh parsley.
> ➤ In a small bowl, whisk together extra virgin olive oil, lemon juice, dried oregano, salt, and pepper to make the dressing.
> ➤ Pour the dressing over the chickpea salad and toss to combine.
> ➤ Serve chilled or at room temperature.

Health Benefits:

> ➤ Chickpeas are rich in plant-based protein and fiber.
> ➤ Cucumber and bell pepper provide hydration and vitamins.
> ➤ Olives and olive oil offer healthy fats and antioxidants.

Preparation Time: 15 minutes

20. Pumpkin Spice Chia Pudding

Ingredients:

> ➤ 1/4 cup chia seeds

- ➤ 1 cup unsweetened almond milk
- ➤ 1/4 cup pumpkin puree
- ➤ 1 tablespoon maple syrup
- ➤ 1/2 teaspoon vanilla extract
- ➤ 1/2 teaspoon ground cinnamon
- ➤ 1/4 teaspoon ground ginger
- ➤ 1/4 teaspoon ground nutmeg
- ➤ 1/8 teaspoon ground cloves
- ➤ Coconut whipped cream for garnish (optional)

Instructions:

- ➤ In a bowl, whisk together chia seeds, almond milk, pumpkin puree, maple syrup, vanilla extract, ground cinnamon, ground ginger, ground nutmeg, and ground cloves.
- ➤ Cover and refrigerate for at least 2 hours or overnight, until the mixture thickens into a pudding-like consistency.
- ➤ Stir the chia seed pudding to redistribute the seeds evenly.
- ➤ Serve chilled, topped with coconut whipped cream if desired.

Health Benefits:

- ➤ Chia seeds are rich in omega-3 fatty acids, fiber, and antioxidants.
- ➤ Pumpkin puree is high in vitamin A and fiber.
- ➤ Spices like cinnamon, ginger, nutmeg, and cloves add warmth and flavor.

Preparation Time: 5 minutes (plus chilling time)

21. Zucchini Noodles with Pesto

Ingredients:

- ➤ 2 medium zucchinis, spiralized into noodles
- ➤ 1 cup fresh basil leaves
- ➤ 1/4 cup pine nuts
- ➤ 2 tablespoons nutritional yeast
- ➤ 1 clove garlic
- ➤ Juice of 1/2 lemon
- ➤ 2 tablespoons extra virgin olive oil
- ➤ Salt and pepper to taste
- ➤ Cherry tomatoes for garnish (optional)

Instructions:

- ➤ In a food processor, combine basil leaves, pine nuts, nutritional yeast, garlic, lemon juice, and olive oil. Pulse until smooth.
- ➤ In a large skillet, heat the pesto sauce over medium heat.
- ➤ Add zucchini noodles to the skillet and toss to coat evenly with the pesto sauce.
- ➤ Cook for 3-4 minutes until the zucchini noodles are heated through but still crisp.
- ➤ Season with salt and pepper to taste.
- ➤ Serve hot, garnished with cherry tomatoes if desired.

Health Benefits:

- ➤ Zucchini is low in calories and rich in vitamins A and C.
- ➤ Basil provides antioxidants and anti-inflammatory properties.
- ➤ Pine nuts are a good source of healthy fats and protein.

Preparation Time: 15 minutes

Ingredients:

- ➢ 1 cup cooked quinoa
- ➢ 1/2 cup shredded purple cabbage
- ➢ 1/2 cup shredded carrots
- ➢ 1/2 cup diced bell pepper (red, yellow, or orange)
- ➢ 1/4 cup diced red onion
- ➢ 1/4 cup chopped fresh cilantro
- ➢ Juice of 1 lime
- ➢ 2 tablespoons extra virgin olive oil
- ➢ Salt and pepper to taste
- ➢ Hemp seeds for garnish (optional)

Instructions:

- ➢ In a large bowl, combine cooked quinoa, shredded purple cabbage, shredded carrots, diced bell pepper, diced red onion, and chopped fresh cilantro.
- ➢ In a small bowl, whisk together lime juice, extra virgin olive oil, salt, and pepper to make the dressing.
- ➢ Pour the dressing over the quinoa salad and toss to coat evenly.

> Serve chilled or at room temperature, garnished with hemp seeds if desired.

Health Benefits:

> Quinoa provides protein, fiber, and essential amino acids.
> Colorful vegetables offer a variety of vitamins, minerals, and antioxidants.
> Olive oil adds healthy fats and richness.

Preparation Time: 20 minutes

23. Eggplant and Chickpea Tagine

Ingredients:

> 1 large eggplant, diced
> 1 can (15 oz) chickpeas, drained and rinsed
> 1 onion, diced
> 2 cloves garlic, minced
> 1 can (14 oz) diced tomatoes
> 1 cup vegetable broth
> 2 teaspoons ground cumin
> 1 teaspoon ground coriander
> 1 teaspoon ground cinnamon

- ➢ Salt and pepper to taste
- ➢ Fresh parsley for garnish (optional)

Instructions:

- ➢ In a large pot or Dutch oven, sauté diced onion and minced garlic until softened.
- ➢ Add diced eggplant to the pot and cook until slightly browned.
- ➢ Stir in chickpeas, diced tomatoes, vegetable broth, ground cumin, ground coriander, and ground cinnamon.
- ➢ Bring the mixture to a simmer, then reduce heat and cook for 20-25 minutes, stirring occasionally, until the eggplant is tender and the flavors are well combined.
- ➢ Season with salt and pepper to taste.
- ➢ Serve hot, garnished with fresh parsley if desired.

Health Benefits:

- ➢ Eggplant is low in calories and rich in fiber, vitamins, and minerals.
- ➢ Chickpeas provide plant-based protein and fiber.

- ➢ Spices like cumin, coriander, and cinnamon add warmth and flavor.

Preparation Time: 35 minutes

24. Coconut Curry Lentil Soup

Ingredients:

- ➢ 1 cup red lentils, rinsed
- ➢ 1 can (14 oz) coconut milk
- ➢ 1 onion, diced
- ➢ 2 cloves garlic, minced
- ➢ 1 tablespoon curry powder
- ➢ 1 teaspoon ground turmeric
- ➢ 4 cups vegetable broth
- ➢ 2 cups chopped spinach
- ➢ Salt and pepper to taste
- ➢ Fresh cilantro for garnish (optional)

Instructions:

- ➢ In a large pot, sauté diced onion and minced garlic until softened.
- ➢ Add curry powder and ground turmeric to the pot. Cook for another minute until fragrant.

- ➢ Add red lentils, coconut milk, and vegetable broth. Bring to a boil, then reduce heat and simmer for 20-25 minutes, or until lentils are tender.
- ➢ Stir in chopped spinach and cook until wilted.
- ➢ Season with salt and pepper to taste.
- ➢ Serve hot, garnished with fresh cilantro if desired.

Health Benefits:

- ➢ Red lentils are a good source of plant-based protein and fiber.
- ➢ Coconut milk adds creaminess and healthy fats.
- ➢ Spinach provides vitamins, minerals, and antioxidants.

Preparation Time: 30 minutes

25. Cauliflower and Chickpea Tacos

Ingredients:

- ➢ 1 head cauliflower, cut into florets
- ➢ 1 can (15 oz) chickpeas, drained and rinsed
- ➢ 2 tablespoons olive oil
- ➢ 1 teaspoon ground cumin
- ➢ 1 teaspoon chili powder

- ➤ 1/2 teaspoon smoked paprika
- ➤ Salt and pepper to taste
- ➤ Corn tortillas
- ➤ Avocado slices for garnish (optional)
- ➤ Lime wedges for serving (optional)

Instructions:

- ➤ Preheat oven to 400°F (200°C).
- ➤ In a large bowl, toss cauliflower florets and chickpeas with olive oil, ground cumin, chili powder, smoked paprika, salt, and pepper until evenly coated.
- ➤ Spread the seasoned cauliflower and chickpeas in a single layer on a baking sheet.
- ➤ Roast in the preheated oven for 25-30 minutes, or until cauliflower is tender and lightly browned, stirring halfway through.
- ➤ Warm corn tortillas in a skillet or microwave.
- ➤ Assemble tacos by filling each tortilla with roasted cauliflower and chickpeas.
- ➤ Garnish with avocado slices and serve with lime wedges on the side.

Health Benefits:

- ➢ Cauliflower and chickpeas provide fiber, vitamins, and minerals.
- ➢ Spices like cumin, chili powder, and smoked paprika add flavor and may have anti-inflammatory properties.
- ➢ Avocado adds healthy fats and creaminess.

Preparation Time: 35 minutes

26. Ginger Miso Soup

Ingredients:

- ➢ 4 cups vegetable broth
- ➢ 2 tablespoons white miso paste
- ➢ 2-inch piece fresh ginger, thinly sliced
- ➢ 2 cloves garlic, minced
- ➢ 2 green onions, thinly sliced
- ➢ 1 cup sliced mushrooms
- ➢ 1 cup chopped kale
- ➢ 1 tablespoon soy sauce or tamari
- ➢ 1 teaspoon sesame oil
- ➢ Cooked brown rice or soba noodles for serving (optional)

Instructions:

> ➢ In a large pot, bring vegetable broth to a simmer over medium heat.

> ➢ In a small bowl, whisk together white miso paste and a ladleful of hot broth until smooth.

> ➢ Add sliced ginger, minced garlic, sliced green onions, and sliced mushrooms to the pot. Simmer for 5-7 minutes until flavors are infused.

> ➢ Stir in chopped kale and simmer for another 2-3 minutes until kale is tender.

> ➢ Remove the pot from heat and stir in soy sauce or tamari and sesame oil.

> ➢ Serve hot, with cooked brown rice or soba noodles if desired.

Health Benefits:

> ➢ Miso paste is rich in probiotics and adds savory flavor.

> ➢ Ginger and garlic have anti-inflammatory and immune-boosting properties.

> ➢ Mushrooms and kale provide vitamins, minerals, and antioxidants.

Preparation Time: 20 minutes

27. Stuffed Bell Peppers

Ingredients:

- 4 large bell peppers, halved and seeds removed
- 1 cup cooked quinoa or rice
- 1 can (15 oz) black beans, drained and rinsed
- 1 cup corn kernels
- 1 cup diced tomatoes
- 1/2 cup diced onion
- 2 cloves garlic, minced
- 1 teaspoon ground cumin
- 1 teaspoon chili powder
- Salt and pepper to taste
- Vegan cheese for topping (optional)
- Fresh cilantro for garnish (optional)

Instructions:

- Preheat oven to 375°F (190°C).
- In a large skillet, sauté diced onion and minced garlic until softened.
- Add cooked quinoa or rice, black beans, corn kernels, diced tomatoes, ground cumin, chili powder,

salt, and pepper to the skillet. Cook for 5-7 minutes until heated through.

> Stuff each bell pepper half with the quinoa and bean mixture.

> Place stuffed bell peppers in a baking dish. Cover with foil and bake for 25-30 minutes, or until peppers are tender.

> If using vegan cheese, sprinkle it over the stuffed peppers during the last 5 minutes of baking.

> Garnish with fresh cilantro before serving.

Health Benefits:

> Bell peppers are rich in vitamin C and antioxidants.

> Quinoa or rice and black beans provide protein, fiber, and essential nutrients.

> Corn adds natural sweetness and fiber.

Preparation Time: 45 minutes

28. Mediterranean Chickpea Wraps

Ingredients:

> 1 can (15 oz) chickpeas, drained and rinsed

> 1/4 cup diced red onion

- 1/4 cup diced cucumber
- 1/4 cup diced tomato
- 2 tablespoons chopped fresh parsley
- Juice of 1/2 lemon
- 2 tablespoons extra virgin olive oil
- Salt and pepper to taste
- Whole grain wraps or lettuce leaves
- Hummus for spreading
- Sliced avocado for garnish (optional)

Instructions:

- In a large bowl, combine chickpeas, diced red onion, diced cucumber, diced tomato, chopped fresh parsley, lemon juice, extra virgin olive oil, salt, and pepper. Mix well.
- Warm whole grain wraps or lettuce leaves in the microwave or on a skillet.
- Spread a layer of hummus on each wrap or lettuce leaf.
- Spoon the chickpea mixture onto the wraps or lettuce leaves.
- Top with sliced avocado if desired.

> Roll up the wraps or fold the lettuce leaves to enclose the filling.
> Serve immediately.

Health Benefits:

> Chickpeas are rich in plant-based protein and fiber.
> Mediterranean vegetables like red onion, cucumber, and tomato provide vitamins, minerals, and antioxidants.
> Olive oil adds heart-healthy fats and flavor.

Preparation Time: 15 minutes

29. Spicy Thai Peanut Noodles

Ingredients:

> 8 oz rice noodles
> 1/4 cup creamy peanut butter
> 2 tablespoons soy sauce or tamari
> 1 tablespoon maple syrup
> 1 tablespoon rice vinegar
> 1 clove garlic, minced
> 1 teaspoon grated ginger

- ➢ 1/2 teaspoon sriracha or chili garlic sauce (adjust to taste)
- ➢ 1/4 cup water (more as needed)
- ➢ 2 cups thinly sliced mixed vegetables (bell pepper, carrot, cabbage, broccoli)
- ➢ 2 green onions, thinly sliced
- ➢ Chopped peanuts for garnish (optional)
- ➢ Fresh cilantro for garnish (optional)
- ➢ Lime wedges for serving (optional)

Instructions:

- ➢ Cook rice noodles according to package instructions. Drain and set aside.
- ➢ In a small bowl, whisk together peanut butter, soy sauce or tamari, maple syrup, rice vinegar, minced garlic, grated ginger, sriracha or chili garlic sauce, and water until smooth. Adjust water as needed to reach desired consistency.
- ➢ In a large skillet or wok, stir-fry mixed vegetables over medium-high heat until tender-crisp.
- ➢ Add cooked rice noodles and peanut sauce to the skillet. Toss to coat evenly and heat through.

- ➢ Garnish with sliced green onions, chopped peanuts, and fresh cilantro.
- ➢ Serve hot, with lime wedges on the side.

Health Benefits:

- ➢ Rice noodles are gluten-free and provide carbohydrates for energy.
- ➢ Peanut butter adds protein, healthy fats, and flavor.
- ➢ Mixed vegetables offer vitamins, minerals, and antioxidants.

Preparation Time: 30 minutes

30. Berry Spinach Salad with Balsamic Dressing

Ingredients:

- ➢ 4 cups baby spinach
- ➢ 1 cup mixed berries (strawberries, blueberries, raspberries)
- ➢ 1/4 cup sliced almonds
- ➢ 1/4 cup crumbled feta cheese (optional)
- ➢ 2 tablespoons balsamic vinegar
- ➢ 1 tablespoon extra virgin olive oil

- ➢ 1 teaspoon Dijon mustard
- ➢ 1 teaspoon maple syrup
- ➢ Salt and pepper to taste

Instructions:

- ➢ In a large bowl, combine baby spinach, mixed berries, sliced almonds, and crumbled feta cheese, if using.
- ➢ In a small bowl, whisk together balsamic vinegar, extra virgin olive oil, Dijon mustard, maple syrup, salt, and pepper to make the dressing.
- ➢ Pour the dressing over the salad and toss to coat evenly.
- ➢ Serve immediately.

Health Benefits:

- ➢ Baby spinach is rich in vitamins A, C, and K, as well as iron and folate.
- ➢ Berries provide antioxidants, fiber, and vitamins.
- ➢ Almonds add crunch and healthy fats.

Preparation Time: 10 minutes

31. Turmeric Cauliflower Rice

Ingredients:

- 1 head cauliflower, grated into rice-like texture
- 1 tablespoon coconut oil
- 1 teaspoon ground turmeric
- 1/2 teaspoon ground cumin
- 1/2 teaspoon ground coriander
- Salt and pepper to taste
- Fresh cilantro for garnish (optional)

Instructions:

- Heat coconut oil in a large skillet over medium heat.
- Add grated cauliflower to the skillet and sauté for 5-7 minutes until tender.
- Stir in ground turmeric, ground cumin, and ground coriander. Cook for another 2-3 minutes until fragrant.
- Season with salt and pepper to taste.
- Garnish with fresh cilantro before serving.

Health Benefits: Cauliflower is low in calories and carbohydrates and rich in vitamins C and K.

➢ Turmeric has anti-inflammatory properties due to its active compound, curcumin.

➢ Cumin and coriander add flavor and may aid digestion.

Preparation Time: 15 minutes

32. Butternut Squash Soup

Ingredients:

➢ 1 medium butternut squash, peeled, seeded, and diced

➢ 1 onion, diced

➢ 2 cloves garlic, minced

➢ 4 cups vegetable broth

➢ 1/2 teaspoon ground ginger

➢ 1/2 teaspoon ground cinnamon

➢ Pinch of nutmeg

➢ Salt and pepper to taste

➢ Coconut cream for garnish (optional)

➢ Fresh thyme for garnish (optional)

Instructions: In a large pot, sauté diced onion and minced garlic until softened.

- Add diced butternut squash to the pot along with vegetable broth, ground ginger, ground cinnamon, and a pinch of nutmeg.
- Bring the mixture to a boil, then reduce heat and simmer for 20-25 minutes until the butternut squash is tender.
- Use an immersion blender to puree the soup until smooth. Alternatively, transfer the soup to a blender and blend until smooth.
- Season with salt and pepper to taste.
- Serve hot, garnished with a drizzle of coconut cream and fresh thyme if desired.

Health Benefits:

- Butternut squash is rich in vitamins A and C, as well as fiber.
- Ginger and cinnamon add warmth and flavor while offering anti-inflammatory properties.
- Coconut cream adds creaminess and healthy fats.

Preparation Time: 40 minutes

33. Lemon Herb Roasted Brussels Sprouts

Ingredients:

- ➢ 1 lb Brussels sprouts, trimmed and halved
- ➢ 2 tablespoons olive oil
- ➢ 2 cloves garlic, minced
- ➢ Zest and juice of 1 lemon
- ➢ 1 tablespoon chopped fresh thyme
- ➢ Salt and pepper to taste

Instructions:

- ➢ Preheat oven to 400°F (200°C).
- ➢ In a large bowl, toss halved Brussels sprouts with olive oil, minced garlic, lemon zest, lemon juice, chopped fresh thyme, salt, and pepper until evenly coated.
- ➢ Spread the Brussels sprouts in a single layer on a baking sheet.
- ➢ Roast in the preheated oven for 20-25 minutes, or until Brussels sprouts are tender and lightly browned, stirring halfway through.
- ➢ Serve hot.

Health Benefits:

- ➤ Brussels sprouts are rich in fiber, vitamins C and K, and antioxidants.
- ➤ Garlic provides immune-boosting compounds and adds flavor.
- ➤ Lemon juice adds brightness and vitamin C.

Preparation Time: 30 minutes

34. Cucumber Avocado Salad

Ingredients:

- ➤ 2 cucumbers, thinly sliced
- ➤ 1 avocado, diced
- ➤ 1/4 cup diced red onion
- ➤ 2 tablespoons chopped fresh dill
- ➤ 2 tablespoons extra virgin olive oil
- ➤ 1 tablespoon apple cider vinegar
- ➤ Salt and pepper to taste

Instructions:

- ➤ In a large bowl, combine thinly sliced cucumbers, diced avocado, diced red onion, and chopped fresh dill.

- ➤ In a small bowl, whisk together extra virgin olive oil, apple cider vinegar, salt, and pepper to make the dressing.
- ➤ Pour the dressing over the cucumber avocado salad and toss to coat evenly.
- ➤ Serve chilled or at room temperature.

Health Benefits:

- ➤ Cucumbers are hydrating and provide vitamins K and C.
- ➤ Avocado adds healthy fats and creaminess.
- ➤ Dill adds flavor and may aid digestion.

Preparation Time: 10 minutes

35. Lentil and Vegetable Curry

Ingredients:

- ➤ 1 cup dried green lentils, rinsed
- ➤ 1 onion, diced
- ➤ 2 cloves garlic, minced
- ➤ 1 tablespoon grated ginger
- ➤ 1 bell pepper, diced
- ➤ 1 zucchini, diced

- 1 carrot, diced
- 1 can (14 oz) diced tomatoes
- 1 can (14 oz) coconut milk
- 2 tablespoons curry powder
- Salt and pepper to taste
- Fresh cilantro for garnish (optional)

Instructions:

- In a large pot, sauté diced onion, minced garlic, and grated ginger until softened.
- Add diced bell pepper, diced zucchini, and diced carrot to the pot. Cook for 5-7 minutes until vegetables are tender.
- Stir in rinsed green lentils, diced tomatoes, coconut milk, and curry powder.
- Bring the mixture to a boil, then reduce heat and simmer for 20-25 minutes, or until lentils are cooked and flavors are well combined.
- Season with salt and pepper to taste.
- Serve hot, garnished with fresh cilantro if desired.

Health Benefits: Lentils are a good source of plant-based protein and fiber.

- ➢ Vegetables provide vitamins, minerals, and antioxidants.
- ➢ Coconut milk adds creaminess and healthy fats.

Preparation Time: 45 minutes

36. Mango Coconut Chia Pudding

Ingredients:

- ➢ 1/4 cup chia seeds
- ➢ 1 cup unsweetened coconut milk
- ➢ 1 ripe mango, peeled and diced
- ➢ 1 tablespoon maple syrup
- ➢ 1/2 teaspoon vanilla extract
- ➢ Shredded coconut for garnish (optional)

Instructions:

- ➢ In a bowl, whisk together chia seeds, coconut milk, maple syrup, and vanilla extract.
- ➢ Cover and refrigerate for at least 2 hours or overnight, until the mixture thickens into a pudding-like consistency.
- ➢ Layer diced mango and chia seed pudding in serving glasses.

➤ Garnish with shredded coconut before serving.

Health Benefits:

➤ Chia seeds are rich in omega-3 fatty acids, fiber, and antioxidants.

➤ Coconut milk adds creaminess and flavor.

➤ Mango provides natural sweetness and vitamins A and C.

Preparation Time: 5 minutes (plus chilling time)

37. Mediterranean Stuffed Portobello Mushrooms

Ingredients:

➤ 4 large portobello mushrooms, stems removed

➤ 1 cup cooked quinoa

➤ 1/2 cup chopped sun-dried tomatoes

➤ 1/4 cup chopped Kalamata olives

➤ 1/4 cup diced red onion

➤ 2 cloves garlic, minced

➤ 2 tablespoons chopped fresh parsley

➤ 2 tablespoons extra virgin olive oil

➤ Juice of 1/2 lemon

➢ Salt and pepper to taste

➢ Vegan feta cheese for topping (optional)

Instructions:

➢ Preheat oven to 400°F (200°C).

➢ In a bowl, combine cooked quinoa, chopped sun-dried tomatoes, chopped Kalamata olives, diced red onion, minced garlic, chopped fresh parsley, extra virgin olive oil, lemon juice, salt, and pepper.

➢ Place portobello mushrooms on a baking sheet, gill side up.

➢ Spoon the quinoa mixture into each mushroom cap.

➢ Bake in the preheated oven for 20-25 minutes, or until mushrooms are tender.

➢ If using vegan feta cheese, sprinkle it over the stuffed mushrooms during the last 5 minutes of baking.

➢ Serve hot.

Health Benefits:

➢ Portobello mushrooms are low in calories and rich in antioxidants and B vitamins.

➢ Quinoa provides protein, fiber, and essential amino acids.

- ➤ Sun-dried tomatoes and Kalamata olives add flavor and nutrients.

Preparation Time: 35 minutes

38. Roasted Root Vegetable Salad

Ingredients:

- ➤ 2 cups diced root vegetables (carrots, parsnips, beets, sweet potatoes)
- ➤ 2 tablespoons olive oil
- ➤ 1 tablespoon balsamic vinegar
- ➤ 1 teaspoon maple syrup
- ➤ 1/2 teaspoon dried thyme
- ➤ Salt and pepper to taste
- ➤ Mixed greens for serving
- ➤ Toasted walnuts for garnish (optional)
- ➤ Vegan goat cheese for garnish (optional)

Instructions:

- ➤ Preheat oven to 400°F (200°C).
- ➤ In a bowl, toss diced root vegetables with olive oil, balsamic vinegar, maple syrup, dried thyme, salt, and pepper until evenly coated.

- Spread the seasoned root vegetables in a single layer on a baking sheet.
- Roast in the preheated oven for 25-30 minutes, or until vegetables are tender and caramelized, stirring halfway through.
- Serve the roasted root vegetables over mixed greens.
- Garnish with toasted walnuts and vegan goat cheese if desired.
- Drizzle with additional balsamic vinegar if desired.

Health Benefits:

- Root vegetables are rich in vitamins, minerals, and fiber.
- Olive oil adds healthy fats and richness.
- Balsamic vinegar and maple syrup add sweetness and flavor.

Preparation Time: 40 minutes

39. Broccoli and Cauliflower Salad

Ingredients:

- 2 cups broccoli florets
- 2 cups cauliflower florets

- ➢ 1/4 cup diced red onion
- ➢ 1/4 cup dried cranberries
- ➢ 1/4 cup sliced almonds
- ➢ 1/4 cup vegan mayonnaise
- ➢ 2 tablespoons apple cider vinegar
- ➢ 1 tablespoon maple syrup
- ➢ Salt and pepper to taste

Instructions:

- ➢ In a large bowl, combine broccoli florets, cauliflower florets, diced red onion, dried cranberries, and sliced almonds.
- ➢ In a small bowl, whisk together vegan mayonnaise, apple cider vinegar, maple syrup, salt, and pepper to make the dressing.
- ➢ Pour the dressing over the broccoli and cauliflower salad and toss to coat evenly.
- ➢ Serve chilled or at room temperature.

Health Benefits:

- ➢ Broccoli and cauliflower are cruciferous vegetables rich in vitamins, minerals, and antioxidants.
- ➢ Dried cranberries add sweetness and fiber.

- ➢ Almonds provide crunch and healthy fats.

Preparation Time: 15 minutes

40. Sweet Potato and Black Bean Quesadillas

Ingredients:

- ➢ 2 medium sweet potatoes, peeled and diced
- ➢ 1 can (15 oz) black beans, drained and rinsed
- ➢ 1/2 cup diced red onion
- ➢ 2 cloves garlic, minced
- ➢ 1 teaspoon ground cumin
- ➢ 1/2 teaspoon chili powder
- ➢ Salt and pepper to taste
- ➢ 4 whole grain tortillas
- ➢ 1 cup shredded vegan cheese
- ➢ Fresh cilantro for garnish (optional)
- ➢ Sliced avocado for serving (optional)

Instructions:

- ➢ Steam or boil diced sweet potatoes until tender. Drain and mash with a fork.
- ➢ In a large skillet, sauté diced red onion and minced garlic until softened.

- ➢ Add mashed sweet potatoes, black beans, ground cumin, chili powder, salt, and pepper to the skillet. Cook for 5-7 minutes until heated through.
- ➢ Lay a tortilla flat and spread a layer of the sweet potato and black bean mixture on half of the tortilla.
- ➢ Sprinkle shredded vegan cheese over the mixture and fold the other half of the tortilla over to cover the filling.
- ➢ Repeat with remaining tortillas and filling.
- ➢ Heat a large skillet or griddle over medium heat. Cook each quesadilla for 2-3 minutes on each side until golden brown and crispy.
- ➢ Slice quesadillas into wedges and serve hot, garnished with fresh cilantro and sliced avocado if desired.

Health Benefits:

- ➢ Sweet potatoes are rich in vitamins A and C, fiber, and antioxidants.
- ➢ Black beans provide plant-based protein, fiber, and essential nutrients.
- ➢ Whole grain tortillas offer complex carbohydrates and fiber.

CONCLUSION

Embarking on a journey toward an Auto-Immune Plant-Based lifestyle is not merely about the food on our plates; it's about nourishing our bodies, minds, and spirits with wholesome, healing ingredients.

Through this cookbook, we've delved into a world of vibrant flavors, nutrient-rich meals, and creative culinary experiences tailored to support your well-being.

As you've explored the pages of this cookbook, you've discovered a plethora of delicious recipes that celebrate the power of plants in promoting health and vitality.

From comforting soups to satisfying salads, hearty mains to delightful desserts, each dish has been thoughtfully crafted to not only tantalize your taste buds but also to nourish your body from within.

By embracing an Auto-Immune Plant-Based diet, you've taken a proactive step towards managing autoimmune conditions and optimizing your overall health. With every meal, you've provided your body with the essential nutrients it needs to thrive, while simultaneously reducing inflammation and supporting your immune system.

But this journey doesn't end here. As you continue to explore the world of Auto-Immune Plant-Based cooking, remember that the kitchen is your sanctuary, and every meal is an opportunity to show yourself love and care.

Experiment with new ingredients, get creative with flavors, and above all, listen to your body's wisdom.

As you savor each bite, may you find joy, fulfillment, and nourishment in every aspect of your Auto-Immune Plant-Based journey.

Here's to vibrant health, delicious meals, and a life filled with abundance.

Cheers to your well-being, today and always.

9 7 9 8 8 8 0 3 7 9 0 0 2